The Ultimate Tinnitus Relief Guide

*How to Cure Tinnitus
For Life with Simple and
Effective Treatments*

Table of Contents

Introduction: What Is Tinnitus and What Causes It?

Tinnitus is a condition that is characterized by swishing, buzzing, ringing, or other similar noises in the head or ear. Although not necessarily a serious or dangerous condition, it can be a symptom of an underlying medical condition and is usually a nuisance. Even though it rarely develops into a serious problem, it can lead to stress, fatigue, sleep problems, memory problems, irritability, anxiety, depression, and concentration difficulty.

Tinnitus can either be objective or subjective. In an objective tinnitus, your doctor may hear the noise while he examines you. In a subjective tinnitus, on the other hand, only you can hear the noise. With treatment, your tinnitus can improve. Anyone can actually get this condition, but some people are more likely to have it than others. For instance, men, adults over sixty-five years of age, people with age-related loss of hearing, and white people are at a higher risk of having it.

Likewise, those who are frequently exposed to loud noises for long periods of time as well as those with post-traumatic stress disorder are more likely to develop tinnitus. All over the world, millions of people are suffering from this condition. In Australia, eighteen percent of adults experience it at some point in their lives. In the United States, around fifty million have it. Other countries where tinnitus is common include the United Kingdom, Canada, Germany, and New Zealand.

Does having tinnitus mean that you are going deaf? Well, it can be a symptom that your hearing system is faulty and may lead to loss of hearing. Then again, it may also be there even if your hearing is perfectly fine. Hence, having tinnitus does not necessarily mean that you are going deaf. However, you should treat it as a warning signal. You should protect your ears against too much loud music or noise. Also, see to it that you visit your doctor once in a while to have your ears checked.

What Causes Tinnitus?

Tinnitus can be caused by numerous factors. Inner ear cell damage, for instance, is one of them. The tiny hairs inside your inner ear move in accordance to the pressure of sound waves. Because of this, your ear cells are triggered to release electric signals to your brain through your auditory nerve. Your brain then interprets such signals as sound. When the hairs in your inner ear get broken or bent, they leak random electric impulses to your brain, which cause tinnitus.

Aside from this, you may also have tinnitus due to other ear problems, conditions or injuries related to the nerves in your ear, and chronic health problems. For many people, tinnitus can also be caused by age-related loss of hearing. You should take note that as you grow older, your hearing gets worse. People above sixty years of age are more prone to hearing loss or presbycusis and tinnitus.

Tinnitus can also be caused by exposure to loud noises for prolonged periods of time. Loud noises, especially those coming from firearms and chainsaws are damaging to hearing. Even portable devices for playing music can cause hearing loss if used excessively. Short-term tinnitus can be caused by short-term exposure to loud concerts while permanent tinnitus can be caused by long-term exposure to loud sounds.

If you are disgusted by your earwax, you should realize that it actually protects your ear canal by slowing down the growth of bacteria and trapping dirt. However, if you have too much of it, you can have a hard time washing it away. This can lead to eardrum irritation or hearing loss, and eventually tinnitus. Similarly, you can have tinnitus if your middle ear bones stiffen or your ear bones grow abnormally.

Nonetheless, tinnitus may also be caused by a variety of other factors, such as Meniere's disease, a condition of the inner ear that involves abnormal inner ear fluid pressure. Tinnitus may also be caused by temperomandibular joint or TMJ disorders in which the joints at the sides of the head are in front of the ears and the lower jawbone meets the skull.

Neck and head trauma can also affect the hearing nerves, inner ear, and brain functioning related to hearing. These injuries, however, only cause tinnitus in one ear. Tinnitus can also be caused by acoustic neuroma, a noncancerous tumor that develops on the cranial nerve and controls hearing and balance. Just like neck and head injuries, this condition only causes tinnitus in one ear.

In rare cases, disorders in your blood vessels can also lead to tinnitus. Neck and head tumors, atherosclerosis, high blood pressure, turbulent blood flow, and malformation of capillaries can lead to pulsatile tinnitus. With atherosclerosis, the cholesterol in your body builds up and the major blood vessels near your inner ear lose their elasticity. This causes your blood flow to be more forceful and makes your ear quicker to detect beats.

High blood pressure can make your tinnitus worse. Hence, you should avoid factors that can increase your blood pressure, such as caffeine, stress, and alcohol. Kinking or narrowing in a vein or artery in your neck can also cause irregular and turbulent blood flow that may lead to tinnitus. Moreover, arteriovenous malformation, a condition in which the connections between the veins and the arteries become abnormal can also cause tinnitus in one ear.

Certain medications can also cause tinnitus. In general, the higher their doses are, the worse they can make the tinnitus. Usually, patients who stop taking such drugs are able to get rid of the unwanted noise in their ears. Some of the medications that are known to cause tinnitus include antibiotics such as neomycin, vancomycin, erythromycin, and polymyxin B, and cancer medications such as vincristine and mechlorethamine. Diuretics or water pills such as ethacrynic acid and bumetanide; quinine medications for malaria, aspirin, and some antidepressants can also cause tinnitus.

Chapter 1: Tests and Diagnosis for Tinnitus

In order for you to find out if you really have tinnitus and how bad your condition is, you need to go to a doctor. The doctor will examine your head, neck, and ears to check for the possible causes of this condition. You will undergo an audiological or hearing exam, movement tests, and imaging tests.

With the auidological exam, you will be asked to sit inside a soundproof room while wearing earphones. Certain sounds will be played into one of your ears at a time. You should let your doctor know if you can hear the sound, so he can compare your test results with those of people with normal hearing.

Your doctor will also require you to clench your jaw, move your eyes, and move your legs, neck, and arms. Such movement tests can help identify any underlying disorder that may need immediate treatment. Furthermore, your doctor will give you imaging tests based on what has caused your tinnitus. You may undergo MRI or CT scans.

Keep in mind that the sounds you hear will let your doctor determine a possible underlying cause for your tinnitus. The muscle contractions in and around your ears can result in sharp clicking sounds that you may hear in bursts. They can last for a few seconds to a few minutes.

Humming and rushing sounds tend to occur when you switch positions or exercise. If you have problems with your blood vessels, such as aneurysm, tumor, high blood pressure, or ear canal blockage, the sound of your heartbeat can be amplified in your ears and you can have pulsatile tinnitus.

As for low-pitched ringing, it may be caused by Meniere's disease. Your tinnitus may be very loud prior to a vertigo attack. On the other hand, you may experience high-pitched ringing if you are exposed to very loud noises or you have had a blow to your ear. Such ringing usually goes away after several hours though.

Then again, if you experience loss of hearing, your tinnitus may become permanent. Other factors that can contribute to the high-pitched ringing that you hear include medications, prolonged exposure to noise, and age-related loss of hearing. Acoustic neuroma can also cause high-pitched ringing in one of your ears.

Furthermore, other factors such as ear canal hair, earwax, and foreign bodies that rub against your eardrum can cause various sounds. Low-pitched sounds may also be caused by otosclerosis or stiff bones in your inner ear. If the cause of your tinnitus is not found, you may discuss certain ways on how you can reduce its severity with your doctor.

Chapter 2: Common Treatments for Tinnitus

In most cases, tinnitus improves over time. However, if your tinnitus is caused by an underlying condition, it can stop or get better once you treat that condition. For instance, if it was caused by an earwax buildup, you can simply have ear irrigation or eardrops to solve your problem. Ear irrigation involves removing the earwax with pressurized water.

If you are not able to identify the cause of your tinnitus, your doctor may recommend a variety of treatments. Although it may never go away, you can still use certain methods to help you manage your condition. If you have lost your hearing at some degree, you need to undergo surgery or resort to using a hearing aid. Otherwise, your condition can get worse. Tinnitus can actually get worse when you strain to listen.

When you correct even a slight hearing loss, your tinnitus will already improve. The part of your brain that is involved in hearing will no longer work as hard, and you will no longer have to pay so much attention to your tinnitus. Your doctor will test your hearing and recommend the necessary treatment. Once you are able to hear better, the audible sounds will override the noises of your tinnitus.

Sound therapy is another ideal treatment option. Tinnitus tends to be more prominent in quieter environments. Hence, you should fill the silence around you with neutral and repetitive sounds so you can be distracted from the noises of your tinnitus. You can turn on the television or radio to provide background noise and drown out the sounds of your tinnitus. You can also listen to natural sounds coming from the sea or rain.

Likewise, you can use a sound generator. It is an electronic device that is similar to a radio and produces quiet, natural sounds that mimic rustling leaves, waves on the shore, or a babbling brook. A white noise generator is also ideal because it produces continuous sounds that are soothing. These devices are recommended to be placed beside your bed so you can listen to them and sleep better.

A lot of people have a hard time sleeping because of their tinnitus. So if you want to fall asleep faster and easier, you should use a sound generator. If you are worried about leaving your device on throughout the night, you should get a model that features a timer so you can set it off at your desired time. This way, you can rest assured that it will turn itself off once you have fallen asleep.

You can also get an ear-level sound generator. It looks like a hearing aid and is recommended to patients with mild to normal hearing loss. If your hearing loss is severe, you can get a hearing aid with a built-in sound generator or a combination instrument.

What's more, you can undergo tinnitus counseling. Most people who suffer from tinnitus have a hard time coping with their condition simply because they do not fully understand it. If you want to know how to manage your condition easily, you should find a hearing therapist, audiologist, or doctor who can administer tinnitus counseling. You will feel much better if you are able to talk about your condition.

Cognitive Behavior Therapy is another popular treatment for tinnitus and a number of other health conditions including post-traumatic stress disorder, anxiety, and depression. It is actually based on the idea that your behavior is affected by your thoughts. So through cognitive behavior therapy, you can successfully change the way you think so you can change the way you behave.

It is also effective in reducing stress and changing the way the patient perceives tinnitus. For instance, if you do not know much about your condition, you may feel depressed and anxious. However, if you begin to understand your condition better, you can find new ways on how you can deal with it on a day to day basis. Changing the way you think about it can really help you learn how you can manage it.

In addition, it can help you learn ways on how to focus your attention away from your problem and take control over your stress. Through cognitive behavior therapy, you can learn how to get rid of negative thoughts and have more positive thoughts. Once you learn to accept the noises, you will be able to live with them more easily. You can have this kind of treatment under clinical psychologists.

You can also undergo Tinnitus Retraining Therapy. It involves relying on your natural ability to adapt to a certain sound so it can become part of your subconscious mind instead of your conscious perception. For instance, you may think that refrigerators, air conditioning units, and electric fans are noisy if you are not used to being around them. However, if you spend more time around these things, the noise they make will eventually be just white noise to your ears.

You will get used to their sounds and you will no longer be disturbed. Tinnitus retraining therapy makes use of a combination of counseling and sound therapy to help you retrain the way your brain perceives tinnitus sounds. It will help you tune out these sounds so you can be less aware of them. This kind of treatment is widely available, although for private use only.

Medications are also recommended, but it should be noted that they cannot really cure tinnitus. They can only help reduce the severity of complications and symptoms. Some of the medications used for treating tinnitus include alprazolam and tricyclic antidepressants, such as nortriptyline and amitriptyline. Such medications can have unpleasant side effects such as dry mouth, constipation, nausea, drowsiness, heart problems, and blurred vision, which is why they are only used for severe tinnitus.

Chapter 3: Alternative Treatments for Tinnitus

Because over-the-counter and prescription drugs are generally not recommended due to their unpleasant side effects, you can use alternative treatments for your tinnitus. Acupuncture, for instance, is very popular. Several studies have found that acupuncture can help improve tinnitus. You should look for an acupuncturist that is knowledgeable and experienced in the field.

Traditional Chinese Medicine can distinguish intermittent or chronic tinnitus from acute tinnitus. Chronic tinnitus is generally characterized by a low buzzing sound and general weakness. Acute tinnitus, on the other hand, is characterized by a low ringing sound and cannot be relived with pressure applied to the ear. A basic acupuncture treatment for tinnitus can last for ten to fifteen sessions.

Hypnosis is another ideal alternative treatment for tinnitus. It can help reduce the distress and negative emotions experienced by the patient. It can also help reduce the sounds associated with the condition. According to one study, seventy-three percent of patients who underwent hypnosis therapy for tinnitus were able to achieve improvement on their condition.

You can also take supplements and B vitamins. Vitamin B12 and zinc are especially recommended. You should take ninety to one hundred and fifty milligrams of zinc everyday for three to six months to improve your condition and if your zinc level is low. A quick way on how you can determine if you are deficient in zinc is if you cannot taste zinc lozenges well.

Researchers have found that zinc is helpful for age-related hearing loss and tinnitus. As for vitamin B12, it is recommended to people who are frequently exposed to loud noises as well as for those who are suffering from loss of hearing or occupational tinnitus. You can take vitamin B12 supplements, but you can also have intramuscular injections weekly to reduce the severity of your tinnitus.

Take note that intramuscular injections can only be availed of at a hospital or clinic. You cannot get them elsewhere. Also, see to it that you find a doctor who can help you administer the injections yourself. Over time, you should learn how to inject your body with the vitamin B12. You should get a prescription for the injectable hydroxycobalamin and syringes.

Another treatment method for tinnitus is Eustachian tube drainage. It is actually a naturopathic technique that is used to provide relief for tinnitus caused by ear, throat, or nose congestion. It works by draining fluid from your ear. You should look for a naturopath to help you learn how to use this treatment method. It is actually fairly easy to do. You can do it to cure a mild ear infection or unlock your ears after diving.

To do this method, you have to open your mouth and look for your back molars using your index finger. Make sure that your hands are clean to avoid infections and other diseases caused by viruses and bacteria. Beyond your molars, you should be able to find the curve of your bones that create a hinge between your lower jaw and upper jaw. Reach for that hinge gently and search for your vertical tendon at the back of your throat. It is actually known as the tonsillar pillar.

Once you found it, you should touch it very gently so you will not gag. Behind it lies your Eustachian tube. It feels like a tiny mole tunnel beneath your flesh. Stroke it gently from the back of your throat towards the middle part or your tongue. You should do this a few times. If your tinnitus is present in both of your ears, you should repeat the process on the other side of your throat.

If you prefer something painless and non-invasive, you can go for neuromodulation using transcranial magnetic stimulation. It is efficient in reducing the symptoms of tinnitus and is actually very popular in the United States and Europe. You can also try Cranio-Sacral therapy. It is a simple yet effective therapy designed to help improve the flow of liquid around the brain and the spinal column. If you work with an experienced therapist, you may only need one session.

Biofeedback is another recommended treatment for tinnitus. It involves the use of mild electrical stimulations to help you notice any physical changes that resulted from stressors. Through this method, you will learn how to put your mind over matter. Biofeedback also involves the use of mechanical noise or background music to avoid having a silent environment. As you know, silence can aggravate tinnitus sounds.

Furthermore, you can try homeopathy. This technique has been around for over two hundred years and involves using plants, minerals, and sometimes even animal materials. If you want to achieve best results, you should work with a trained homeopath. Nonetheless, you can also use herbs and other remedies to make you feel better.

Chapter 4: Vitamins and Herbs for Tinnitus

As mentioned in the previous chapter, certain herbs and vitamins can help treat tinnitus. In fact, herbs and vitamins can help fight the free radicals that damage tissues and ear cells. They can also help alleviate symptoms and improve blood flow. Then again, before you try any herbal remedy, see to it that you consult your doctor to avoid any complications in case you are currently on a particular medication or you have an existing medical condition.

Nonetheless, ginkgo biloba is one of the most recommended herbal remedies for tinnitus. It is known to improve blood flow to the periphery or edges of your body. If your tinnitus is caused by problems in your circulatory system, taking ginkgo biloba can help you. It can even improve your focus and memory. Ideally, you should take two hundred and forty milligrams of ginkgo biloba in a capsule form everyday. Within six weeks, you should be able to find relief. During this time, you can lower your dosage to just forty to sixty milligrams daily.

Aside from ginkgo biloba, you can also try burdock root, bayberry bark, hawthorn leaf, myrrh gum, and goldenseal. These herbs can efficiently counteract any infections as well as purify your blood. You can also use fenugreek seeds to make tea. It can help you find relief for your condition. Likewise, you can use the essential oils of cypress, lemon, rose, and rosemary for massaging or aromatherapy. You can also use them in a vaporizer. These herbs can help improve your blood circulation.

Japanese cornel dogwood is ideal too. It is a small tree that is native to Korea, Japan, and China. According to practitioners of Traditional Chinese Medicine, the fruit of this tree can significantly improve the condition of your kidney, liver, and lower back. It has a potent astringent property. It can even treat deafness, vertigo, impotence, hypertension, and of course, tinnitus.

According to a study published in The American Journal of Chinese Medicine, the ursolic acid found in Japanese cornel dogwood is a powerful antioxidant that can protect damaged ear cells. However, due to its other properties, it may not be advisable for pregnant women and people with diabetes, HIV, and cancer. If you have any of these conditions, you should consult your doctor before using this remedy.

In addition, you can try wolfberry. The wolfberry shrub is thorny and produces red berries. It can also be found in China. Practitioners of Traditional Chinese Medicine usually use these berries to treat liver, kidney, and blood problems. They also use it to treat diabetes, poor eyesight, and other diseases. Such berries are high in antioxidants and essential oils.

According to Penelopy Ody, an herbalist and author of the book The Holistic Herbal Directory, these berries can be mixed with cereal if you do not want to eat them alone. Eating them will help you treat dizziness and tinnitus that are associated with kidney problems. Then again, if you have diabetes or hypertension, you should not take wolfberries along with your medication.

Furthermore, you should keep in mind that it is crucial to have a healthy immune system. Hence, you need to take vitamins and supplements. See to it that you are not deficient in vitamins A, B complex and E. You should also take sufficient doses of zinc, manganese, potassium, magnesium, flavonoids, and pantothenic acids.

Vitamin E, in particular, is very important. You can get it from corn, sunflower, safflower, and soybean. It is a powerful antioxidant that can protect your cell membranes against oxidative stress. In fact, Phyllis Balch and James Balch, authors of the book Prescription for Nutritional Healing, state that vitamin E can increase your blood circulation and help treat hearing loss and tinnitus.

Then again, you should take note that vitamin E is also an anticoagulant, which means that you can have complications if you have blood problems. Make sure that you consult your doctor before you use it.

Chapter 5: Diet and Lifestyle Changes for Treating Tinnitus

Maintaining a healthy diet is critical in the treatment of your tinnitus. If you want to reduce the noises and be able to live normally, you should avoid certain food products. If your tinnitus is caused by an underlying condition, such as high blood pressure, you should avoid foods that can trigger such condition. If you are overweight, you have to lose the excess weight so you can reduce the ringing in your ears.

Foods to Avoid

Salt is among the worse foods that you can eat if you are suffering from tinnitus. Too much salt in your body can restrict your blood vessels, reduce the blood flow to your ears, brain, and eyes, and increase your blood pressure. You should take note that an increase in your blood pressure can aggravate your tinnitus. Hence, you should cut down on salty snacks, such as chips. You should also avoid eating pre-packaged and processed foods because they are high in salt content.

Sugar is another food to avoid if you have tinnitus. Sugar metabolism actually has a significant role when it comes to the functioning of your auditory system. You see, your auditory system and brain do not have an inherent supply of food. They merely rely on the regular delivery of glucose and oxygen in your blood. So when their supply is interrupted or disturbed, you can be at risk of a system damage or imbalance.

Researchers have also found that eighty-four to ninety-two percent of individuals with tinnitus suffer from hyperinsulinemia, a sugar metabolism disorder. It occurs when your body becomes inefficient in delivering sugar to your cells and becomes insensitive to insulin. It is characterized by an increased level of insulin in the blood. Although it is not particularly a dangerous condition, it can lead to type 2 diabetes.

Just like simple carbohydrates and refined sugar, sweeteners and other sugar substitutes can also make your tinnitus worse. They can actually have worse effects than sugar. Hence, you should avoid them at all costs. Aspartame, which is usually found in diet beverages, and glutamate, can act as excitatory neurotransmitters in your brain. They can cause your neurons to fire repeatedly until they die.

When your nervous system gets damaged, you can develop neurodegenerative disorders, such as tinnitus. Moreover, aspartame can lead to weight gain and more cravings for sugar. If you consume too much sweets and carbohydrates-rich foods, you can be at risk of obesity, hypertension, heart diseases, diabetes, and other health problems that can make your tinnitus symptoms worse.

You should also avoid flavor enhancers, especially monosodium glutamate or MSG, which is commonly found in processed food products. Even though the Food and Drug Administration considers MSG to be safe, it is still a type of sodium that can contribute to water retention and affect your inner ear. Also, MSG breaks down in your body as glutamate which serves as an excitatory neurotransmitter and causes your neurons to fire until they die. For a lot of people, glutamate is the main reason why they develop tinnitus.

You see, when the hearing cells in your cochlea are damaged due to noise exposure, medication, or infection, they release excessive amounts of glutamate which floods the neuro-receptors in your auditory pathway. When your neurons die, large amounts of free radicals are also released to your system. So if you do not want your tinnitus to get worse, you should avoid food products that contain MSG or hydrolyzed vegetable protein.

In addition, you should avoid bad fats. Trans-fats and saturated fats, in particular, can have numerous negative effects on your body. Saturated fats are not good for people with hyperinsulinemia and diabetes because they can reduce good cholesterol and increase bad cholesterol in the body. They can also increase triglycerides which can lead to atherosclerosis, a risk factor for stroke and heart disease. It can also reduce blood flow.

If you have tinnitus, you need your blood flow to your inner ear to increase so you can maintain healthy cells and get rid of toxins. Good fats, on the other hand, come in the form of unsaturated fats. These fats can be obtained from fish, vegetables, olive oil, and nuts. They can lower bad cholesterol and increase good cholesterol in your body. They can also lower your blood pressure, increase your energy levels, and reduce inflammation.

Furthermore, you should avoid caffeine and alcohol. Caffeine can be found in tea, coffee, chocolates, and soda. It can stimulate your central nervous system and cause your blood pressure to rise. It can also lead to a number of health problems if consumed at excessive amounts. Ideally, you should not consume more than five hundred milligrams of caffeine per day. If you do, the hair cells in your ears can go into a state of excitotoxicity and destroy the nerve cells in your inner ear. This can lead to tinnitus and hearing loss.

Alcohol, on the other hand, can increase your blood force by dilating blood vessels. This can result in more blood flow to your ears. If you drink too much alcohol, your blood pressure can increase and you can be at a higher risk for tinnitus. If you already have tinnitus, your condition can get worse. If you find it impossible to quit drinking, you should at least do it in moderation.

Men should not consume more than two twelve-ounce bottles of beer, one and a half ounces of distilled spirits, or five ounces of wine per day. Women should consume less alcohol and has to cut the recommended amount of alcohol for men in half.

Lifestyle Changes

Everyone needs to consume vegetables, fruits, whole grains, nuts, and beans. Maintaining a Mediterranean diet is the best way to avoid tinnitus or prevent it from getting worse. This diet involves whole grained pasta or bread, olive oil, yogurt, cheeses, fruits, and vegetables. You need to have servings of these foods everyday. Likewise, you should eat eggs and fish a few times per week. You may also have sweets and red meat occasionally.

Of course, you also need to exercise on a regular basis. Exercising has plenty of benefits. For instance, it can elevate your mood and alleviate your stress. As you know, stress can make your tinnitus worse. Hence, you should find ways on how you can relax and stay healthy. Exercising also keeps your body energetic and in top shape. If you stay sedentary, you can develop various health problems that can make your tinnitus worse. If you are not athletic, you can do simple exercises such as running, walking, or jogging.

You can also practice yoga and other relaxation techniques, such as meditation and guided imagery. Furthermore, you can join a support group or speak with a psychologist. Joining a support group will allow you to share your experiences with people who are also suffering from tinnitus. Being around other people who have the same condition as you can be comforting since you will not feel like an outsider. If you cannot find a support group in your area, you can join a forum on the Internet.

Likewise, you can speak with a psychologist regarding your problems with tinnitus. Counseling can help you ease your burdens and free your mind from worries. Speaking with a professional will also assure you that you are in good hands. Your psychologist can give you advice on how you can live normally with your tinnitus.

Conclusion

Thank you again for downloading this book!

I hope this book was able to help you understand your condition better and learn ways on how you can treat your tinnitus.

The next step is to apply what you have learned in this book. Until you fully apply what you have learned, the information has no power!

Finally, if you enjoyed this book, please take the time to share your thoughts and post a review on Amazon. It'd be greatly appreciated!

Thank you and good luck!